How To Tell Children About Sex

By Clyde M. Narramore Ed.D.

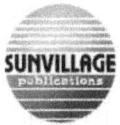

www.sunvillagepublications.com

How To Tell Children About Sex
By Clyde M. Narramore

Copyright © 2010

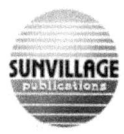

SUNVILLAGE
publications

www.sunvillagepublications.com

Cover design by www.WebCopyAlchemy.com

INTRODUCTION

In this volume, *How to Tell Your Children About Sex,* Dr. Clyde Narramore offers more than sex instruction. He effectively shows that attitudes are among the most important considerations in wholesome sex education.

Many parents and teachers of yesterday failed to realize the importance of instructing their children in matters of sex. Today's parents, however, have come to realize that wholesome sex education, or the lack of it, affects a person as long as he lives. It affects his attitudes. It colors his life. It helps to determine how he will react to his environment. It determines what kind of a parent he will become.

The development of wholesome attitudes entails more than an understanding of the basic facts of the anatomy and physiology of reproduction. Dr. Narramore presents in this book a much-needed, sound and spiritual treatment. It will guide adults in the important job of providing wholesome sex education at the time when it will do most good for the development of a mature, well-balanced person.

RICHARD A. CROSSE, M.D.

Huntington Memorial Hospital
Pasadena, California

ACKNOWLEDGMENTS

Several people have made important contributions to this book. I wish to express special appreciation to Dr. Richard Crosse, Alice Elliott, Marion Ferguson, Sylvia Locke and Georgiana Walker.

Grateful appreciation is expressed to my wife, Ruth, for her months of planning, research, writing and editing.

CONTENTS

The Meaning of Sex 9
Ask Yourself 11
Why Tell Your Child? 14
Is Information Dangerous? 17
When Should Sex Education Begin? 20
Guides in Sex Education 23
The Right Vocabulary! 27
Modesty in Young Children 29
Family Dressing and Undressing 33
Curiosity 36
Children's Early Questions 40
How Much Should a Child Be Told? 43
Learning from Nature 45
The New Baby Brother or Sister 48
When Children Share Information 55
Experimentation 58
Sharing Beds and Bedrooms 62
Children Who Do Not Ask... 64
Teasing... 69
Facts about Masturbation 72
"Bad" Language 76
Helping Children Accept Their Roles 79
Should a Child Be Given Books about Sex?..... 83
Explaining the Father's Role in Reproduction.... 86
When Children Ask about Menstruation 90
The Preadolescent and His Questions 92
Safeguarding Your Child 96

The Meaning of Sex

Have you ever thought of the various meanings that people attach to the word "sex"? It signals something different to every person. To one it is sacred and holy. To another it is "terrific." To someone else it may seem sordid, and to yet another it is a silent, "hush-hush" subject.

Sex can also mean confusion, sorrow and embarrassment. Why? There are many reasons. Many of them stem from childhood. Our parents and grandparents may have had somewhat prudish ideas concerning sex. To them the subject was often taboo. So yesterday's children frequently received untruthful and evasive answers. It is not difficult, then, to understand why people who have come from this kind of background may feel uncomfortable and uneasy when their own children ask direct questions.

Alice and John are a fine, sincere young couple who want their children to have a clear, wholesome understanding of sex matters. Yet for them it isn't easy. Even the children's simplest questions make John and Alice blush with embarrassment. John puts it this way: "When I was a boy the word 'sex' wasn't spoken in our home." Alice's background was much the same. So even though they are now adults, it is hard for them to overcome the marks left by their early training. That is why they are uncomfortable when they need to discuss these things with their children.

Here is an interesting fact: We can tell our children how a tree grows — or what makes it snow — or why a car needs gasoline. But to explain about ourselves, how we began, how our bodies function — well, that is different. And in a way, it should be. Because "sex" is indeed something special. It is so closely intermingled with our emotions and intense feelings that it would be unnatural and inappropriate to talk about it in the same offhanded manner in which we would the weather.

Yes, sex education includes more than anatomical facts. It takes in attitudes, personal example and manner of living. These impress a child as much or more than facts. And it is fitting that they should.

Most parents have a sincere desire to give their children a good beginning in all phases of life. This includes wholesome attitudes toward sex — a most important part of living.

When your child becomes an adult, what will the word "sex" mean to him? Naturally, that's up to *you.* Your skill in sex education today will determine his feelings tomorrow. You carry the key to his future!

Ask Yourself

It is hard to help your children if you need help yourself. That is why it is so important to analyze *your own attitudes.* Your feelings about sex subtly but definitely influence your entire approach. Therefore, it is wise to take a close look at how *you* feel.

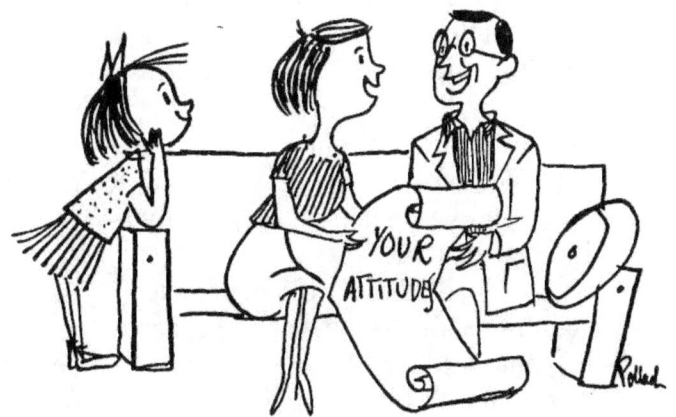

It is important to analyze your own attitudes because they subtly but definitely influence your child's feelings.

The following questions are designed to help you evaluate your own attitudes.

1. Do you shy away from the sex questions your children ask?   Yes   No

2. Do you think fathers should answer the boys' questions and mothers, the girls'? Yes No
3. Did (or does) diaper changing and toilet training seem distasteful to you? Yes No
4. Do you feel that talking to your child about sex matters will cause him to become too curious and lead to experimentation? Yes No
5. Are you discreet in your conversation about matters of sex? Yes No
6. Do expressions of affection embarrass you? Yes No
7. Do you often feel annoyed with the opposite sex? Yes No
8. Are you ever ashamed of your own interest in sex? Yes No
9. Do you still have difficulty under standing some of the sexual aspects of your childhood? Yes No
10. Can you talk rather freely and with ease on matters of sex education? Yes No
11. Do you think specific terms such as "urine," "penis" and "vagina" should be used in talking to children about their bodies? Yes No
12. Do you and your mate feel free to discuss your sex problems and rela-tionships? Yes No

13. Would "you prefer giving your child a
    book on sex rather than talking with
    him?   Yes   No

How do you rate? Are there certain attitudes you
need to improve?   Although it is not essential to
have a perfect score, the answers below are undoubtedly the most desirable ones.

Questions 1-4, 6-9 and 13 —No
Questions 5 and 10-12 —Yes

Why Tell Your Child?

During a series of parent meetings at the church, the pastor stressed the importance of Christian sex education. "It is our sacred responsibility," he said, "to help our sons and daughters develop into well-adjusted Christian men and women."

The pastor was right. Christ-centered sex education *is* important and these are some of the basic reasons.

1. Sex education helps a child to wholesomely accept each part of his body and each phase of his growth. It enables him to discuss physical development without shame and embarrassment.

2. Sex education helps a child to understand and be satisfied with his role in life. Boys grow to be men and fathers. Girls grow to be ladies and mothers.

3. Sex education erases unhealthy curiosity. It takes away the mystery. Children who understand the facts and who know that their parents will truthfully discuss their questions have no cause for worry or concern. They are not attracted to dirty stories and pornographic material. Sex education does not keep children from wanting to know —but it *does* eliminate the need for secretive investigations and unfortunate experiences.

4. Wholesome information guards against serious

complexes and maladjustments later on in life. It encourages a child to develop *normal* attitudes. Childhood misinterpretations and fears carry over into adulthood and often produce twisted, abnormal patterns in later life.

5. Sex education with a Christian viewpoint helps a person spiritually. It clears his mind of distracting sex questions. It fosters a deep respect for God and His plan of human development.

6. Sex education builds a child's confidence in his parents. If mothers and fathers are honest and helpful regarding matters of sex, children learn to also trust and confide in them about many other things.

7. Sex education given at home in dignity and authority tends to overcome and nullify the un wholesome information that reaches boys and girls from outside sources.

8. Sex education makes human reproduction clear and wholesome. A child should feel that having children is right. He needs to know, as shown in Genesis 1:24, that God planned for each living creature to bring forth after its kind.

9. Sex education provides a child with sound knowledge and good attitudes which pave the way for him to happily accept new brothers and sisters. New family members are not considered "mysterious intruders."

10. Sex education, while making a child proud

of his own sex, will help him appreciate the attributes and capacities of the opposite sex.

11. Sex education removes many sources of fear. It assures a person of his own capabilities and normalcy.

12. Sex education strengthens a person's self-confidence. It helps him feel comfortable and well poised around others. This is true regardless of a person's age.

13. Sex education enables a young person reaching adulthood to make sound, mature decisions about courtship and marriage.

14. Sex education lays the groundwork that helps to build a solid marriage. Young people who enter marriage with mature, wholesome attitudes and understanding are beginning on a sound premise.

15. Sex education prepares a child to later be come a parent who can, in turn, comfortably teach his own children. Most parents who find it difficult to discuss sex matters with their children were raised in homes where there was little or no proper sex education.

Is Information Dangerous?

Mr. Martin was a little worried over his wife's direct answers to the questions their children asked about sex. He felt that such frankness might invite trouble. These possibilities loomed in his mind: "Do sex facts shock children? Does sex education cause undue curiosity?"

Mr. Martin is not the only one who wonders about these things. Many adults are concerned about how children may react to sex information. But those who have thought it through realize that wholesome sex education does not shock children. It is a normal part of living. Youngsters accept sex information with a wholesome, matter-of-fact attitude when it is presented naturally and without much ado. Knowing the truth is less disturbing than *not* knowing the facts and wondering what they are.

Another significant fact is that *sex experimentation comes most frequently from a child who is uninformed.* In fact, experimentation is one means of getting information. Clearly stated answers take away from a child's need for finding out on his own. Children who have a wholesome understanding of human development find it much easier to control themselves. Several research studies show that the

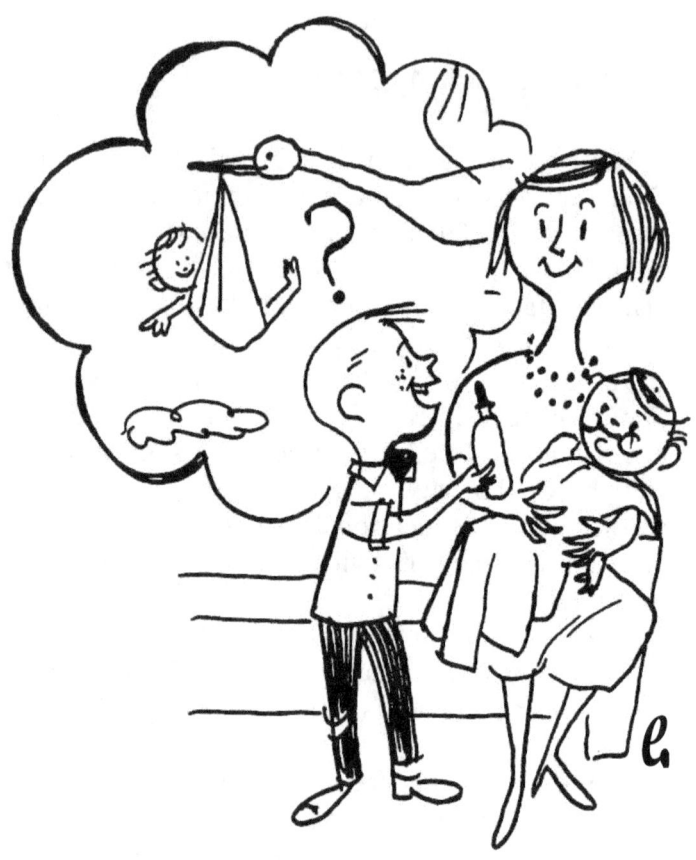

Children accept sex information with a wholesome, matter-of-fact attitude when it is presented naturally and without much ado.

18

typical sex offender usually comes from a home where he has received little or no sex education.

Unwholesome curiosity is *not* the result of sex education. On the contrary, children who know the facts and who realize that their parents are willing to talk with them are less preoccupied with sex matters than are other children who are un-informed. Informed children still have healthy in-quisitiveness; they still ask questions — but they direct their questions to their parents.

Naturally, there are some sensible guides in giving sex education to a child. Too much information may bewilder and trouble a child. Some parents un-wisely tell all they know. The child is often confused and overstimulated when his sex learning comes in such large doses. Listen to the child's question. Tell him the thing he wants to know. That's probably all he is interested in for the time being. Frank and simple answers are always in order. Then wait patiently for the next question. It may be weeks later before he asks again —but he will.

You can save your child from embarrassment and criticism if you tell him that sex matters are to be discussed *at home.* Explain to him that other parents want to talk to their own children about such things. Let him know that although you, his parents, are willing to discuss any question with him, other adults may not want to do so. Your child will readily accept these few simple rules. And it will keep him from pulling "boners."

When Should Sex Education Begin?

Not long ago a friend and I were talking about family living. During our conversation he asked, "When do you think parents should start giving their children sex education?"

"Well, Don," I said, "parents are giving their children *some* kind of sex education all the time — whether they realize it or not."

Yes, a child's sex education begins the day he is born! You love him, care for him, play with him and laugh with him. When he is hungry you feed him. When he is dirty and wet, you clean him and make him comfortable. Is this sex education? Yes, indirectly it is. Through these loving acts you introduce him to a world of love. You give him his start toward being a warm, friendly person, capable of trusting and loving others.

Your mature, matter-of-fact attitude toward diapers, bathing and toileting shows your child that body functions are normal and right. All of this forms the setting and background for the innocent little questions he asks later on. Even though the child is young, he senses your attitudes and he begins to develop his feelings around yours.

"But," you may ask, "when is the best time to give a child sex information?"

The answer is simple. Tell him when he becomes

curious — when he starts to ask questions. This usually begins somewhere between the ages of two and four. By this time your child is talkative and active. The "great big world" looms before him. And he asks questions — about *everything.* Naturally, he is interested in himself — in his own body. And of course he notices the body differences of the people with whom he lives and plays.

Parents often say to me, "Dr. Narramore, do you know of a good book about sex education? Our boy (or girl) is nearly thirteen and we want to tell him the facts of life."

Questions like this would be humorous if they weren't so unfortunate. Evidently these parents do not realize that they have been giving their children sex education for years. The very fact that they have not talked with them tells these children that sex is something to avoid discussing. And, of course, thirteen years of age is much too late to begin. By then, some of the most important and most impressive years of life have already passed.

When a child raises questions, do not put off your discussion until a more "convenient time." If you do, the questions may be forgotten and the time of natural interest will be gone.

Sometimes more is actually involved than the specific question might imply. When parents alert themselves to a child's *interest* and *wonderings* they may discover that the unstated questions need discussing, too.

Some children ask questions surprisingly early. And these first "whys" and "whats" are the outgrowth of a youngster's natural curiosity. A very young child is likely to notice sex differences in his own family. He sees that Mommie looks different from Daddy. If there are sisters and brothers, he soon realizes that little girls are made differently from little boys. "Why?" is a natural question. A simple, honest answer reassures the child that differences are normal—that God made girls one way—boys another, and that both are "right" for them.

Unanswered questions at this time may leave a young child with serious worries. He may think that his sister has lost a part of herself, and that his own penis might disappear. A little later, perhaps at three, four or five a child raises questions about his own beginnings. "Where did I come from?" he asks. "How do babies get born?" As he grows older he may not remember having even asked many of these questions. But the attitudes he picked up from you will remain — possibly a lifetime.

Questions are your cues. When a youngster begins to ask, it is your responsibility (and privilege) to help him understand the God-planned wonders of life!

Guides in Sex Education

1. *The Environment* — Sex education develops best in a sweet, Christian environment. Not long ago my wife and I visited in the home of a lovely Christian family. It was a pleasant evening. The family atmosphere was just "right" — wholesome and relaxed. I noticed the easy, cordial relationships be tween the parents and the children. It is this kind of climate that nurtures good sex attitudes.

2. *Examples* — Children unconsciously absorb the attitudes and feelings of their parents. In other words, a good example is one of the best teachers.

3. *Embarrassment* — Obvious embarrassment on the parent's part can signal the child not to ask questions. Or it may cause him to seek information outside the home — information that is unwholesome and unchristian.

4. *Questions* — Your child's normal curiosity shows up in the form of questions. This is good. He is interested in everything he sees — including himself. And he wants to know the answers.

5. *Birds and Bees* — Children can learn about birth, growth and development from pets. A mother cat with baby kittens, or a mother dog and her puppies are fine demonstrators. However, some parents and teachers talk about animals in order to avoid dis-

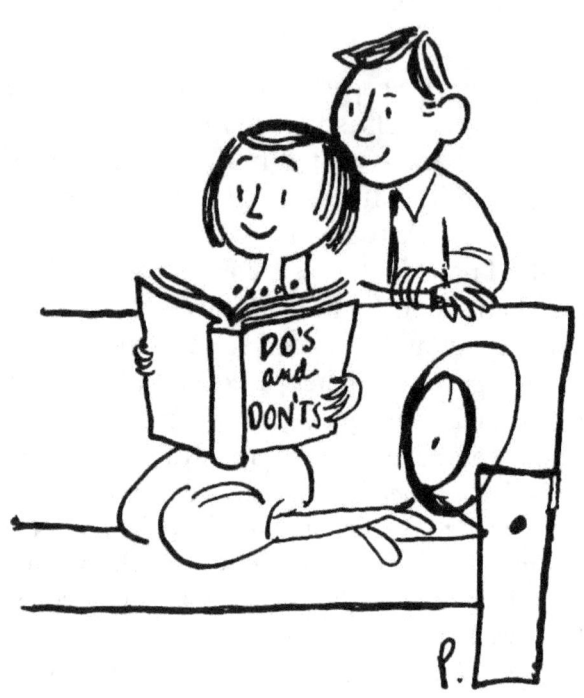

A few basic guides will serve you well.

cussing human beings.   But evading an issue never settles it.   Children want to know about *people.*

6. *Timing* — As children grow and observe people around them,   they   naturally   become   curious.   So wait for your cues.   It is unwise to rush your child into sex education.

7. *Listening* — Listen attentively to your child so you will know what he is really asking.   A parent who both hears and speaks can usually uncover a child's misconceptions.

8. *Why Wait— Now* is the time.   When a child asks, he is ready to learn.   So don't try to divert the youngster's attention.   He'll wonder why you don't want to tell him.

9. *Too Much* — Answer your child's questions, but don't go beyond his   level of interest or under standing.   Too   much   information   confuses   the answer.

10. *Relaxed —A* child learns best when he is at ease.   It will help if you preface your remarks with, "I'm glad you asked."

11. *No Lectures* — Sex education is not a lecture; it is a process.   It begins when a child is tiny and continues until he grows to adulthood.   Don't wait until your son or daughter approaches adolescence, then call him in for a lecture on the "facts of life." Rather, talk with him whenever he wants to know.

12. *Attitudes* — Your attitude is just as important as your answer.   Your child may forget what you say, but he will always remember your attitude.

13. *Yourself* — Children can pick up sex information almost anywhere — playmates, adults, books, television, radio and many other places. But the best place to gain wholesome information and healthy attitudes is from *you*. It is *your* responsibility. Don't leave it up to your school or church. Use this privilege *yourself.*

14. *Living* — Sex education is not separate from other areas of life. It should be handled as any other aspect of living. It does not require a "special time" and a "special place." It "grows" with the child and should be learned just as naturally as any other phase of development.

The Right Vocabulary!

During baby's first year he makes many exciting discoveries — his hands, his toes, his hair, his ears. Soon he can identify these parts of his body by name.

Knowing the right names for *all* parts of the body is an important aspect of sex education. The right names may seem difficult, although they may seem that way more often to the parents than to the child. But just as Junior quickly learns elbow, ankle and forehead from hearing the names spoken — so he will learn penis, testicle, buttocks, anus, vulva and vagina if his parents use these terms as they talk with him. The words are not hard to say, and they should be used with accuracy when speaking with a child about his body or when answering his questions.

A youngster needs these words. Asking questions will be easier if he has the words to say what he means. Furthermore, if he learns the correct terms in the beginning, he won't have to relearn them later.

Names for body functions are important, too. Children learn many of them in everyday living. Eating, hearing, digesting, lifting, speaking — these all explain body functions.

We call it sex education when the occasion arises to use words such as urinating or menstruating. It would be easier if these words were easier to say. But since there are no accurate substitutes, it is better for a child to learn the right terms at home.

No doubt your child will use simple words of his own choosing for everyday use. This is all right. But be sure that you use the correct terms often enough for him to know what each word means.

As with all sex matters, it is best to teach a young child that with the exception of asking to go to the bathroom, toilet words and really "personal words" should be used only in his own home or with his own parents. It is an important part of his personality development to learn what is socially acceptable — and what is not.

Modesty in Young Children

Three-year-old Betty was *unusually* quiet. Mother looked out of the kitchen window into the back yard. What she saw made her groan, half in laughter and half in despair! But Betty was perfectly happy. All of her clothes were off — again. And she was holding the garden hose high over her curly head, letting little trickles of water sprinkle down over her chubby little self.

Will she ever have any modesty? her mother wondered. But Betty's mother had no need for worry. Modesty does come.

Just "growing up" and wanting to act like other people will teach this small nudist to be modest. There is no set time when this happens, but sometime between the ages of six and eight a child begins objecting to being seen without his clothes. He wants the bathroom door closed when he is toileting. He closes the door to his room, or jumps into the closet if you come into his room unexpectedly.

You can help your child develop modesty by respecting this new desire for privacy. Encourage other members of the family to let him close doors without teasing him. Explain that he has individual rights, even though he is young.

The development of modesty in a child is not

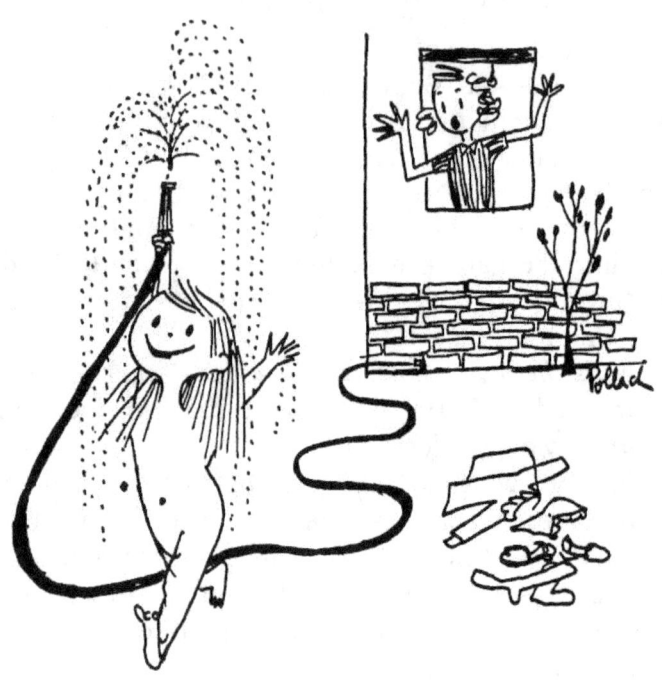

Just growing up and wanting to act like other people will teach a young nudist to be more modest.

entirely related to his ideas on sex. He becomes modest as he grows conscious of being a separate, real little person — himself! The seven- or eight-year-old enjoys short times of being *apart* or *alone*. He slips away from the family to work on a project; or he closes the door to his room to look over his treasures. He also likes to get into and out of his clothes without anyone around. This means that he is "growing up." It is an important part of his personality development — and it is basic to wholesome modesty.

On the other hand, children are *taught* modesty — both by instruction and by example. It is *not* something that is entirely instinctive. The naked savage does not understand modesty; it is not in his culture. And your children will not understand modesty either — *until they are taught.*

Small children must be told what is proper and what is not. And they must be given reasons for the restrictions placed on them. Tell them *why* they must not dress and undress in front of windows. Tell them *why* they must not do their toileting outside in the yard. Little girls should be told what is "lady-like" — to keep their dresses down. Little boys must learn what is expected of them —to keep their pants up and to keep them fastened. Children can learn that it is "nicer" to whisper when they need to go to the bathroom. They will understand *why* when you explain that this is of no concern to others. There is much that children must learn. And they *will* learn —in time. But it takes patience and repeated instruction on your part. And like other social graces and good manners, it will finally be absorbed.

But it does little good to "preach" modesty if you do not practice it yourself. Many adults are *not* modest, much to their own shame and the embarrassment of others.

Once when a little boy was eating his supper in the kitchen with the baby sitter, his mother, who was going out for the evening, came to kiss him good-by. She was dressed in an ultra modern, low-cut evening gown.

"Where are you going, Mommie?" asked the child.

"To a concert, dear."

The boy looked worried. "But somebody might *see* you!" he said.

And he was right. Modesty begins by example. And we as parents should set that example.

But there is a "happy medium." It is unwise for parents to make *too* much of modesty. As children grow older they naturally develop normal attitudes about propriety. And parents who *overemphasize* modesty only cause their children to gain peculiar and false attitudes about themselves and others.

Family Dressing and Undressing

Living in a family means living close to each other. And it is only natural that there are times when family members see each other dressing and undressing. Although each one has some privacy, occasionally a child will come into a room and find brother or sister, or father or mother not fully dressed. When this does happen, remember that your calm, poised attitude means more than anything else you can possibly say or do. For example, a child may forget what you tell him, but more than likely he will never forget your attitude. Your naturalness and your poise let your child know that the human body which God has created is wholesome and worthy of dignity.

When "Teddy" suddenly comes into a room where either his mother or father is not fully dressed, the parent can say, "Hi, Teddy. I guess I didn't close the door, did I? Would you please hand me my robe?" This takes care of the situation without making the child feel uncomfortable. If you can be at ease it will keep him from becoming embarrassed about his own body. And he will learn to accept himself in a relaxed, wholesome manner.

However, in our society a healthy respect for privacy is important. And although a youngster

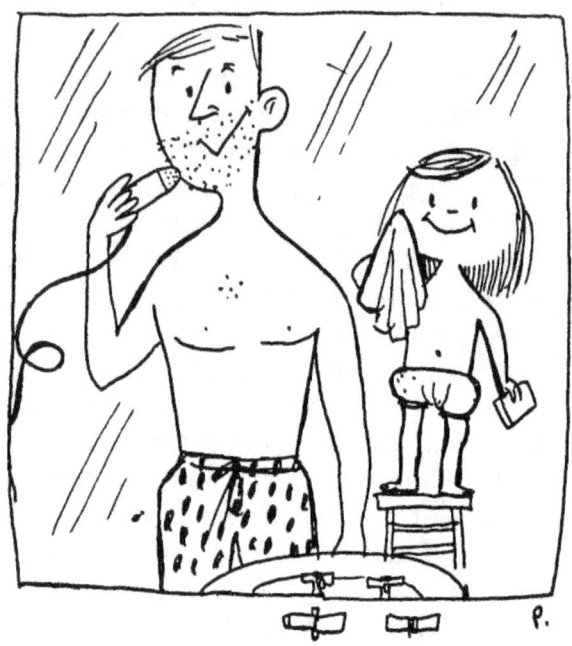

Your naturalness and poise let your child know that the human body which God has created is wholesome and worthy of dignity.

learns about an adult body from an occasional glimpse of his parents without their clothes, it is not well for a child to be constantly exposed to adults who are not dressed.

Seeing a naked body too frequently may arouse feelings and emotions too strong for a child to cope with — feelings beyond his understanding. It is good to plan your living with a fair amount of privacy — but with a willingness to accept any family intrusion with a matter-of-fact attitude.

Curiosity

Curiosity is the very beginning of learning. Parents are pleased when children want to see . . . to touch . . . to taste. "Look again," they say, holding little Johnny a bit closer.

And he looks — because a child's curiosity is unlimited. He wants to know about the world around him. He wants to know about himself —and naturally, he wants to know about matters of sex, too. Youngsters know how their own bodies look. But they wonder about others: "Are other children made like 1 am? What do bigger people look like?"

How can such curiosity be handled in a way that will help a child to learn and at the same time keep his behavior socially acceptable? Children are as *wholesomely* curious about sex as they are about airplanes, animals and boats. Their curiosity about their bodies is normal and natural. And when parents realize this they find it easy to help their children.

Families with both boys and girls have many natural ways in which the children can be brought together. Toileting, bathing and dressing are normal times to see and learn. Wise parents do not keep children apart because they are inquisitive; rather, they provide wholesome, supervised *together-times* to satisfy young curiosities.

I remember Mr. and Mrs. "Smith" who handled their little boy's curiosity most unwisely. His first grade teacher reported that Jimmie had been overly interested in the little girls. Several times he had "peeked*' in the rest-room and had tried to get one or two of the girls to show him how they looked without panties.

The Smiths were shocked and embarrassed to think their son would behave in such a way. So they asked me to visit their home and discuss Jimmie's problem with them. When I did, their *own* attitudes came to light.

"Well, Dr. Narramore," Mrs. Smith said with alarm, "I don't know what makes Jimmie act the way he does. Why, even at home when I change his baby sister's diapers, he wants to see what's going on"

"Have you ever let him see?" I asked.

"Of course not," she replied. "Whenever I change her diapers or give her a bath I always lock the door so he can't get in!"

This, of course, was *not* the solution. If Jimmie had seen his little sister being bathed and changed, his curiosity would have been satisfied and he probably would not have resorted to such objectionable behavior at school.

But what if there is no sister or brother? There are still other ways. Try visiting a relative or a neighbor who has a baby. Just the everyday bath and routine diaper changing will give your child an

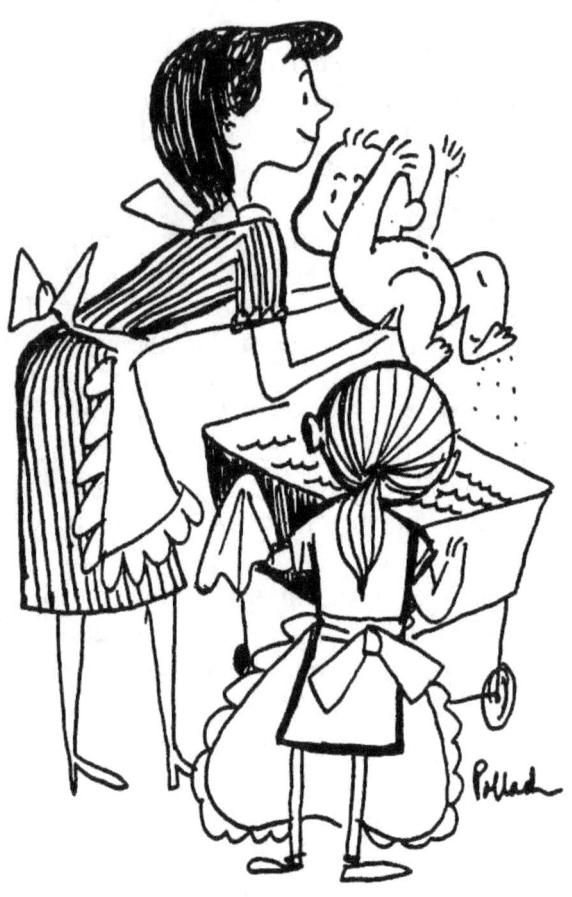

*Children are as wholesomely curious about sex as
they are about airplanes, animals and boats.*

opportunity to see another body, and to gain knowledge through seeing.

Some parents occasionally let their own dressing time, toilet time, or bath provide the opportunity for the youngsters to see an adult undressed. If you can comfortably do this at one time or another it will give your child a chance to satisfy his curiosity in a perfectly natural way.

However, you may be surprised! Your child may not seem to notice —or he may walk into the bathroom talking about the new slide on the playground, or about the cut on his knee. In your eagerness to help your child learn, remember: Sex is only one of the many interests in his busy mind!

Children's Early Questions

Children have boundless curiosities! They want to know about everything — bugs, stars, water, trains, paint, mud, worms— and a child also wants to know about himself.

"What's that?" a small child asks, pointing to his genitals. If the small inquirer is a boy, the mother (or father) might answer, "That is your penis. All boys and men have one."

If the questioner is a little girl, you might say, "That is your vulva; all girls and mommies are made that way."

But a child's curiosity does not stop with his own body. "Where is Mary's penis?" young Bub asks, remembering how sister looked when Mommie popped both of them into the bathtub last night.

Questions concerning basic sex differences must be answered clearly to assure the child that he is made the way he should be. You might say, "Boys and girls are always made differently. God planned it that way. All boys have a penis; girls do not. You are made just the way God wanted you to be."

A child is likely to repeat questions concerning sex differences. Be patient. If a youngster repeats a question, he simply needs to hear the answer again.

The child may be only three or four when he starts

wondering about his beginnings. His reasoning powers are beginning to develop. He remembers the day he went with Daddy to the pet shop and bought their wiggly puppy. On another day he was with Susie and her mother when they stopped in the dime store to get a goldfish. "Mommie," he asks, "Where did you get me?"

Your answer is important. And it must be truthful. In time there will be many more questions related to babies and sex.

Truthful answers to these first questions build a happy and firm foundation for future information. The stork story, or some other evasive untruth can only lead to mistrust and doubt. Sooner or later your child will learn that you have not dealt with him honestly.

"Where did I come from?" the three-year-old asks.

Mother smiles. "You grew right inside of mother's body, and when you were big enough you were born."

"Tell me some more, Mommie," he may say. So you repeat it.

He may not fully understand, but he feels happy and satisfied. Soon he will ask other questions.

"How do babies get out?" This question may or may not arise at the same time a youngster asks where babies come from. You can tell your child, "Babies come out of a special opening in the mother's body. It is between the upper part of her legs."

Children are often confused and do not understand that in a girl or a woman there are two different openings. It is helpful if you explain, when it seems natural to do so, that in front of the vagina is another opening for urination. It is called the urethra.

"Does it hurt to have a baby?" Be truthful, but cheerful. "It may hurt some, but a mother is so happy to see her new baby that she soon forgets any pain. Doctors know how to make mothers comfortable. Mothers go to the hospital when babies are born because they need extra care, not because they are sick."

"Do daddies have babies inside of them, too?"

"No, only mommies do. God did not make any place in a man's body for a baby to grow. That's the way God planned it."

"Will I have a baby?" Most children, both boys and girls, ask this. Tell them, "Yes, when you grow up and get married you can have babies." Help small boys to realize that they will be daddies, that they will work and care for the mother and the children.

How Much Should a Child Be Told?

You have heard the old saying, "Things are seldom what they seem." In a sense, questions about sex are not always what *they* seem. For example, when little Johnnie asked his parents where he came from, he did not have the slightest thought about sex. He had heard the other children tell which state they were born in and he merely wanted to get his own birthplace straight. "Was it Kansas or Missouri?"

It is possible to tell your child too much about sex —more than he really wants to know. This is why *listening* is as important as explaining.

Listen carefully to what your child asks. Fortunately he does not want or need a lengthy, technical lecture. Furthermore, a simple, honest answer is more easily understood.

You can easily tell when a youngster's curiosity is satisfied. If there are no more questions — if he starts looking for his baseball — or if he asks for a peanut butter sandwich, you can be sure he has all of the information he wants or needs just now.

It has been said that an adult can talk about sex for hours, but a small child's interest usually lasts for about thirty seconds! Too much information is bewildering and confusing. It can also stimulate a child's interest too early.

The amount you tell a child depends partly upon his age. Very young children do not understand much about causes, results and implications. For example, a child of three may ask, "Where do babies come from?"

You might answer, "They grow inside the mother until they are big enough to live in the outside world." To a child approximately four or five years old you might add, "All children come from then-parents — from their mother and daddy. Each baby starts as a tiny little baby inside the mother. Then it grows and grows until it is big enough to live outside the mother."

As a child grows older he will ask more about the same questions. *Some parents make the mistake of reading their own adult understanding into the child's question.* But to go too deeply into this is neither wise nor necessary.

Learning from Nature

Debbie and her mother were over visiting a neighbor lady who asked, "Debbie, would you like to see our baby kittens?"

"Oh, yes," replied Debbie, jumping up and down.

So they went out to the back porch. And there they were! All five little fuzz balls, nestled up to their Mommie for a nice warm "lunch."

"But, Mommie," asked Debbie, "what are they doing? Eating their mother?"

"No, honey," the mother answered. "They are nursing. You see, when kittens are tiny, they suck warm milk from the mother cat. All babies nurse. God causes the milk to come into the mother's breast so that the babies will have just the food they need. When the babies grow old enough to *drink* instead of suck, they will not need to nurse anymore. Then the mother's milk will go away."

And so Debbie learned how baby kittens nurse from their mother. But she also learned that baby boys and baby girls nurse from their mother or from a nice warm bottle.

Learning from nature is helpful to a child. And children should be encouraged to do so. But *learning from nature never takes the place of a child learning about himself.*

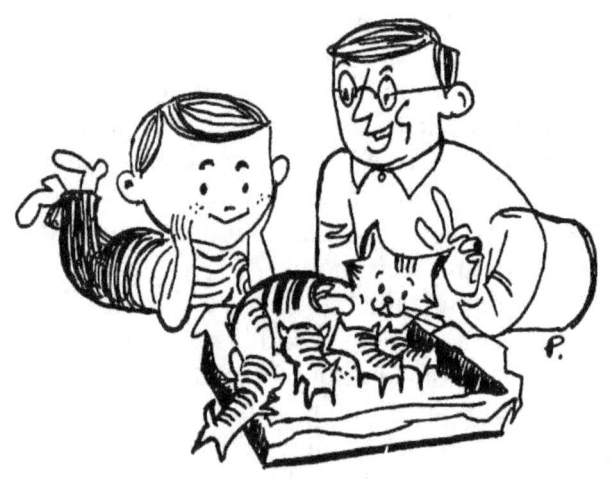

Learning from nature is helpful, hut it cannot take the place of a child learning about himself.

A young child's curiosity begins with his own body, or differences between himself and others. He may also wonder where babies come from. Explanations about birds, bees and flowers do offer a way to avoid direct answers, but they are so remote from the real interest that they may *confuse* rather than *inform*.

An older child is interested and impressed with the intricate ways God planned for the reproduction of plants, insects and all living things. Differences as well as similarities become fascinating information for the inquiring mind of the older preadolescent and the adolescent child. But these understandings need to be based on a wholesome knowledge of human sex facts.

It is not unusual for a child who sees animals mating to also ask questions about people. This gives parents an excellent opportunity to point out that like baby colts, calves and other animals, children, too, have both a mother and a father. If a child asks if parents "mate," a mother or father can explain that they *do* but that they are different from animals. Parents can explain that mothers and fathers love each other with all their hearts. That is why they get married and live together —so that they can have a happy family and raise the children whom they love. Such explanations help children understand the mutual and tender love of parents. These explanations also use a natural interest that children have in animals and turn it into wholesome instruction regarding people.

The New Baby Brother or Sister

Getting ready for a new baby — what a happy time this can be for all the family! And what's more, the anticipation and joy over the expected "newcomer" also offers many splendid opportunities for brothers and sisters to gain a basic understanding of human beginnings. There is much preparation needed to welcome this new member of the family. Layette? Yes, but more than that. Parents should talk over the coming event with the brothers and sisters. Then-lives will be affected by the "little one," too.

This is no time for surprises. An unannounced baby can cause misunderstandings and even serious emotional damage. Children must be made ready to accept a new brother or sister.

Bobbie proved this point. A few years ago I was called upon to give psychological help to this five-year-old boy. He refused to speak. Although he had attended kindergarten for several months, he never uttered a word in public.

One day I visited his home. Suspecting that Bobbie had been the victim of a traumatic experience, I asked his parents if he had ever been shocked or terribly frightened.

"Yes," replied the father. "It happened when he was about two years old. That's when his younger brother was born. My wife was about eight months

48

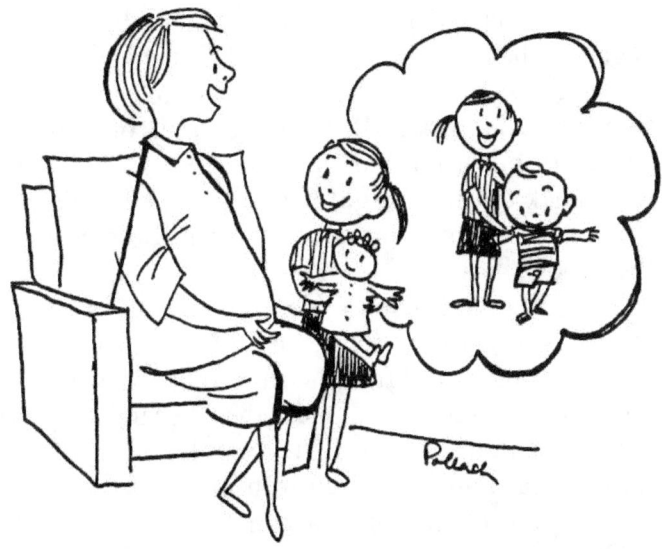

*Your child will be more ready to welcome the
new baby if he knows just what to expect.*

along. I'll never forget that night. She and I had been talking about when we should tell Bobbie that he was to have a new brother or sister. We didn't know just how to go about it, but we decided we would tell him the next morning. Well, the next morning was too late, because that night my wife began to have labor pains and I rushed her to the hospital. Then I dashed back home, picked up Bobbie, who was still sleeping, and took him to some friends of mine in a nearby town. Then I went back to the hospital where I spent the night."

"Was it the next morning when Bobbie received the shock?" I asked.

"Yes," he continued. "You see, he never roused from his sleep that night, and when he awoke the next morning my friends said that he screamed violently for several minutes, then became sick. He wasn't acquainted with the people, so he didn't know what had happened to him."

"Has he spoken since that time?"

"No, hardly any. He understands, and hears us, but just won't talk."

After careful diagnosis we worked with Bobbie and within a year he was talking and reacting in a normal fashion.

Bobbie's case is both extreme and unusual. But it illustrates the effect of shock on the human body and on the emotions.

Parents who "surprise" their children with a new baby may not injure them this severely. But they *do* make it difficult for them to fully understand and to accept the newcomer.

"Where did he come from?" "Are they telling me the truth?" "They like him better than they do me/' "Why does Mommie want to hold that little baby all of the time?"

These are natural reactions for children who are not sufficiently informed. Such feelings spell trouble for your child, and for the new baby, too. Jealousy and dislike rush to the mind of the youngster who un-expectedly finds a tiny "darling" in his mother's arms.

Parents may think that the other children in the family just naturally know that a baby is coming. "I'm so big!" Mother laughs. "How can they help but know? We talk about it a lot."

But the change comes gradually. And young children may not pay much attention to grown-up conversation. As a result, they may not fully under-stand. This is good to a certain point, because it is extremely hard for a youngster to have the seemingly endless wait of seven or eight long months. But after a little while, the parents should break the happy news that a new brother or sister is coming to live with them.

Sometimes children do notice that mother is getting larger. "Mommy, you're so fat," says three-year-old Mark. "Mother is a fatty — Mother is a fatty," sings four-year-old Joy.

Now is the time for honesty. "Yes," mother agrees,

"I *am* getting bigger. And there's a good reason why Mommie's tummy is getting larger. Let me tell you a very happy secret: A little baby is growing inside of me!" Then as you give the children a little hug, add: "This is just the way I looked when I was waiting for you to be born. I was happy *then* and of course I'm happy now."

Children enjoy getting things ready for the new baby. They like to see the tiny new clothes and they take pride in folding them and putting them away. The more the child is in on the "getting-ready," the more he feels that this is *his* baby, too.

If the new baby is going to use the crib now being used by an older child, be sure to make a special occasion of getting the larger bed all ready before you say much about using the crib for the new baby. This will help the older child share happily. In fact, some parents have asked where they should let the new baby sleep. Often the youngest child suggests that the newcomer use *his* crib!

Your youngster will be more ready to welcome the new baby if he knows just what to expect. These are some of the things that a child needs to know:

—We do not know whether the new baby will be a boy or a girl. But we are sure that God will send the one that is *just right* for the family.

—New babies are little. Show him just about how big, about like Susan's doll — so little that they can't play games or talk.

—New babies can't eat grown-up foods. They
have no teeth.

—Babies suck to get their food. Mother's breasts
will have milk in them when the baby is ready
to eat. (Let him know he also nursed.)

—A new baby cries often, but it doesn't mean
he is hurt or sick. Crying is his way of talking.
He is letting you know that he wants some
thing to eat, or some dry clothes.

—The new baby will sleep much of the time.
Babies need lots of sleep to help them grow.

Your child should also know ahead of time that
Mother will be going to the hospital. He will be
interested in the whole plan: who will stay with
him — how long Mother will be gone — how much
fun it will be for Mother to come home and see the
family again. All of these facts can be woven into a
happy bedtime story. And telling it once is not
enough. It is a story your child will want you to
repeat quite often. When you prepare him in this way,
he will be at ease when the time comes for Mother to
leave for the hospital.

During the time of waiting for the new baby,
children ask many things. You can expect questions
such as these more than once:

—"Does the baby hurt you?"

—"Is the baby in your stomach now?"

—"How did the baby get inside?"

—"How is the baby going to get out?"

— "Is it going to hurt you when the baby comes out?"

The age and the understanding of your child will tell you how much information is needed to satisfactorily answer his questions. Be truthful, keeping in mind that each basic fact will strengthen your child's understanding. Smile as you answer. Be happy and make the little questioner comfortable and happy. Remember: Your wholesome, Christian attitude toward sex will become his! You may have to repeat things you thought he clearly grasped, but these repetitions are important — someday he will fit all of the pieces of information together and *really* understand!

When Children Share Information

After a Bible story and bedtime prayers, Mother tucked Janie in for the night. Just as Mother was ready to leave the room, Janie propped herself up on one elbow and said, "Mother, do you know what? Linda says her mother is going to have a baby. She even told me how it was going to be born."

Janie's mother felt a waver of uncertainty. *Should children be talking about such things?* she wondered.

Parents are often alarmed when they learn that their children have been "talking things over." But one thing is certain: Some such talk among children is inevitable, and not all of the childish exchange of information is bad or unwholesome. In many cases it is of real value — because children explain things to each other in a natural, easy manner and in language they understand.

If you have a friendly, relaxed relationship with your children, built on years of working things out together, you can expect them to bring bits of picked up information for you to explain. This is an invaluable opportunity: a time for you to correct mistaken ideas, a time for you to minimize anxieties and a chance to explain things further.

What should parents do when children share sex information? Because of the nature of sex, children

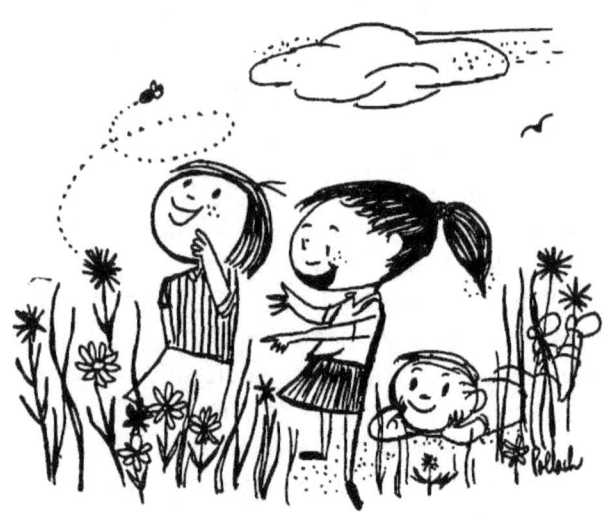

In many cases, childhood sharing of information may have real value because children explain things to each other in a natural, easy manner and in language they understand.

do need guidance. Be sure your child knows that most parents want to tell their *own* youngsters about sex matters. Explain that you, too, prefer that questions and ideas about sex be discussed *at home.* Help him understand that there are many times when a conversation about sex is out of place —that these subjects are usually discussed just in the privacy of the family.

Children need to learn what is acceptable and what is not. Naturally, young children do not know what *is* appropriate unless you tell them. It is your responsibility to quietly explain *why* we talk about sex matters in a discreet manner. Such instruction not only teaches a child to be more acceptable during his formative years; it also helps him to be discreet when he becomes an adult. We all know grownups who are shunned because they have never learned that sex matters are personal — not to be glibly spoken about like the weather.

When children share sex information, you have at least two responsibilities: (1) Explain to your child why we do not discuss personal matters out of the home, and (2) explain to your child that the boy or girl who continually talks about sex is not using good manners and probably does not have the right information anyway. Assure your child that you will be glad to talk with him (or her) about personal matters anytime he wants to.

Experimentation

On a number of occasions, school officials have asked me to assist them in working with parents on problems concerning sex play among small children. Although most of these incidents have taken place in the neighborhood and not at school, disturbed parents have reported the occurrence to school principals and teachers, asking that their child not be permitted "to play with such children."

Many mothers and fathers have been shocked and upset to find a group of neighborhood children involved in sex play. But there is no real need for panic. Sex play and experimentation are not at all uncommon among children between the ages of four to ten.

Youngsters want to compare, to find out. So behind closed doors they show each other their buttocks and genitals. They experiment with different ways to urinate. Girls stand up — boys sit down. They giggle about toilet activities and bathroom words. Sometimes their play is more subtle —and they play operation, doctor and nurse. Sometimes it is more extreme — and the child becomes anxious and a bit frightened.

Little girls often play mother. "I have a baby growing inside of me," announces five-year-old

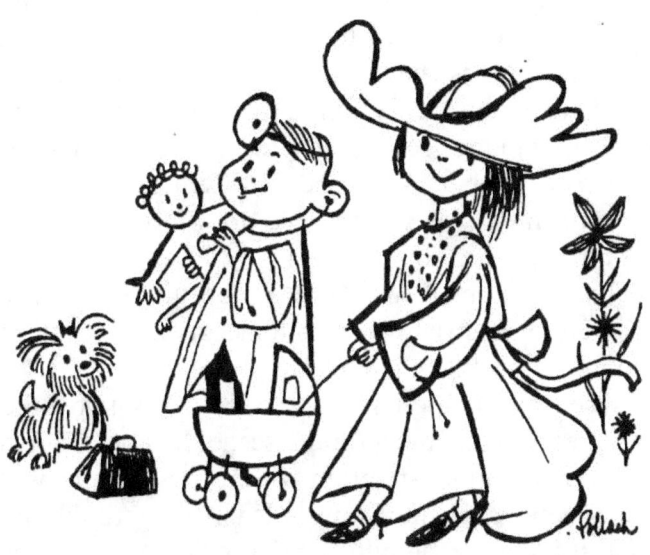

Sex play and experimentation are not uncommon among young children. Sometimes it is more subtle —playing "operation," "doctor' and "nurse"

Peggy. Little boys have grown up feelings, too. "I'm a fireman." Answers Tommy, "and I haven't any time for babies, I've got to put out a fire."

Occasionally, parents are so shocked when they find children have been engaged in sex play that they forbid their child to ever play with the group again. But this is seldom the solution. Such "solitary" punishment may only emphasize the incident and make it stand out unhappily in the child's memory as a *dirty* and *bad* experience. Remember: *Whole some attitudes toward sex are not built on feelings of guilt and shame.*

The best thing you can do is to quietly talk with your child, answer his questions, give explanations and minimize the whole affair.

Wise parents step in and lead children to other activities — without causing a scene. It is not difficult to divert a child's attention if you present him with some new and interesting ideas. Try stimulating interest in other activities by providing some new materials and making a game out of it.

Children must learn what is acceptable behavior. So be loving —but be firm. A definite "no" will put an end to undesirable play. And do not waver or show uncertainty when you say "no." A child *welcomes* definite limits. He feels safe when he knows that his parents are interested enough in him to set up rules.

When you hear of young children experimenting

with sex play, you can remember that some of it is a natural part of growing up. On the other hand it might be their way of saying, "We have questions in our minds about sex, but no one is giving us wholesome sex education."

Sharing Beds and Bedrooms

"The house is just too small!" is a lament in many homes today. And it is an honest worry because it is difficult to successfully juggle a growing family into too few bedrooms.

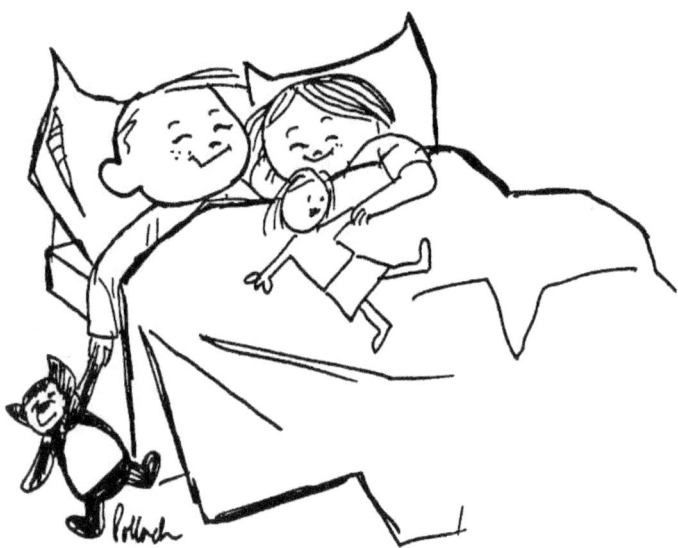

Children who share a bed regularly are subject to physical contacts that may lead to sex play.

Parents wonder, "Should the children share beds or bedrooms?" "How long can the baby sleep in our room?"

Every child should have his own bed. Youngsters who regularly share a bed cannot avoid physical contacts that invite sex play. Although in every child's life there is usually some such play without any harm, invitation to such activities must be avoided whenever possible.

As I counsel with adults who have sex problems, I find that a significant number of them trace their initial sex experiences to times when they slept with brothers and sisters or with relatives or other friends. Sex feelings are real, even to children. And undue stimulation can arouse and awaken sex feelings that are difficult to control. Many well-meaning parents would be surprised if they knew the amount of sex play and masturbation that takes place when children are forced to sleep together.

If it can be managed, brothers and sisters should have separate rooms after the age of five or six. If this is impossible, use your ingenuity to give each child as much privacy as possible. Furniture already in your home can be arranged to give each child an area of his own. Book shelves, chests of drawers and desks make good semi-partitions.

Children should not be required to share a room with their parents. Even little ones become alarmed and afraid when they become aware of the intimacies of their parents. Darkness is no real protection since children have sharp ears and active imaginations. Even if it means a nightly unfolding of the living room sofa, it is well worth the effort to give parents and children the privacy they need.

Children Who Do Not Ask

It was refreshment time following a meeting of the mother's group at church. Two of the ladies were chatting when one said, "What do you tell your children when they ask about sex? Ronnie has been pestering the life out of me lately with all sorts of personal questions. And frankly, I don't know how much I should tell him."

"That's not *my* problem," her friend answered. "Linda never asks *anything*. It worries me a little because she simply never says a word. It isn't natural."

Like Linda, some school age children have never asked about sex. And in a way it is unfortunate because early questions are usually easy ones — easy, but vitally important. -Parents who share the basic and simple facts of sex with young children have paved the way for more complex questions later on.

Why are some youngsters so silent? There may be a number of reasons. Their interest may not be stimulated through natural events in family living. The *only* child, the *last* child in the family, or a youngster whose brother or sister is born when he can't remember the event, is not alerted by the "new baby." So his curiosity may be lacking.

Sometimes the child who does not ask about sex is trying to be "good." Perhaps he has picked up the impression that questions about his body are bad. Such a situation develops when the parents are very strict about all behavior. You have heard parents say, "Why did you do that, don't you want to be *good?"* Children who are under constant pressure to be "good" hesitate to ask questions. They are afraid to risk parental disapproval by making a needless mistake.

The child who is overanxious can best be helped by relaxing the pressure. Praise the youngster for his accomplishments — even though they may seem relatively insignificant. Make your rules less rigid; put your child at ease. Plan fun times with him. Be generous with your smiles and affection. When he begins to feel confident and relaxed with you, he will be less afraid to share his curiosity and his questions.

Sometimes the child who does not ask, has already done so — outside the family circle. But he may have been embarrassed or rebuffed. As a result, he does not feel free to raise further questions — *anywhere.*

Children may remain silent for various reasons — known and unknown. But regardless of the reason, children who never ask the usual questions about human reproduction need help just as much as those who do.

There are many ways you can help your child

develop normal interests in personal matters. It may be through his pets. Animals provide valuable object lessons. Many children are encouraged to ask about the beginnings of life through the birth of new kittens or puppies, or by observing these "babies" nurse. But although animals are fine, they are not enough. Your child is entitled to understand *himself.* The knowledge he gains from animal life must be transferred so that he will also learn about *human beginnings.*

Sometimes a few well-chosen books will induce good questions. These books do not necessarily need to be ones that you definitely consider as sex education. They can be delightful stories which can easily lead to a conversation about new babies and where they come from. Your librarian can suggest suitable reading materials for your child.

Another "question-raiser" is the new baby himself. So when your friend or neighbor has a newcomer, take your child with you to visit the little one. You need not say anything especially. Just let your child see the tiny new fellow. And don't worry—the wheels of curiosity will soon start to turn. You can help things along by making statements such as, "You were just about that size when you were born."

In other words, be a good teacher. Set the stage so that your child finds himself in a situation where asking questions is a natural sequence.

But suppose your child is old enough to attend

school and still isn't asking questions, even when it seems he has every reason to ask. What then? Is it hopeless? No, you can still help him. Try to *sense* his unasked questions. Observe his behavior closely enough so that you know what his interests are. Then start from there.

Sometimes a child's silence does not indicate a lack of interest, but rather, a fear of asking. When a child senses a grownup's embarrassment or a tendency to avoid such subjects, he often gets the idea that he should not raise questions. So he keeps quiet.

But if time goes on and your child never opens the subject himself, you can help him by beginning the discussion in a natural and straightforward way.

"Did you know that Aunt Hazel and Uncle Jim are going to have a baby? You know, when I was very small I wasn't sure just where babies came from. Have you ever wondered, honey? When you were little, what did *you* think?"

Asking a child what he *used* to think may make it easier for him to express his ideas. In this way he won't have to admit what he is thinking now. You can help guide the conversation by saying, "Of course, you and I know that the baby is growing inside Aunt Hazel's body. All babies grow inside their mothers."

There are other ways of approaching the subject, too. As a mother you can choose some quiet, happy time — perhaps after evening prayers — and then say to your child, "I'm so glad we have you. I can remember before you were born. I used to wonder if you would be a little boy or a little girl. But I didn't really care which you were —I was just happy that a baby was growing inside of me. Every time I'd feel you moving around I'd think, 'This baby feels like a nice healthy little fellow.'"

Your loving, relaxed discussion assures your youngster that any questions or ideas he may have are acceptable to you. Let him hear some of the friendly, neighborhood news that mothers and fathers exchange. "Mrs. Benson is at the Memorial Hospital. She has a new baby boy." "Did you know the Johnstons are going to have another baby? Perhaps it will be a girl this time. They already have four boys."

So if your child does not raise the usual questions, use your ingenuity. If you are alert you will soon find many opportunities (and *natural* ones) to encourage him to "talk things over."

Teasing

When Dad arrived home from work he noticed his little girl, June, playing in the yard with the neighbor boy who had moved in across the street. An hour later when the family gathered around the supper table Dad came out with, "Well, Junie, who's your new boy friend?"

Uncertain as to just what Dad meant, June squirmed a little and remained silent.

"Come on now," Dad teased, "tell us who your boy friend is. I saw you playing with him this afternoon."

June, half embarrassed, glanced at her mother, then noticed her brothers and sisters giggling as they began to chime in with the chorus: "Junie has a boy friend, Junie has a boy friend."

Teasing about "boy friends" and "girl friends" is quite common — especially among parents who have not thought it through. "Harmless," you say. Yes, in a way. But something all intelligent parents want to consider carefully.

When a child is continually teased about such a playmate, he soon learns to be embarrassed and uncomfortable. It doesn't take much teasing to make him feel ill at ease and strange about playing and associating with *all* playmates of the opposite sex.

When children have been teased, they sometimes say, "I don't like boys," or "I don't like girls." This,

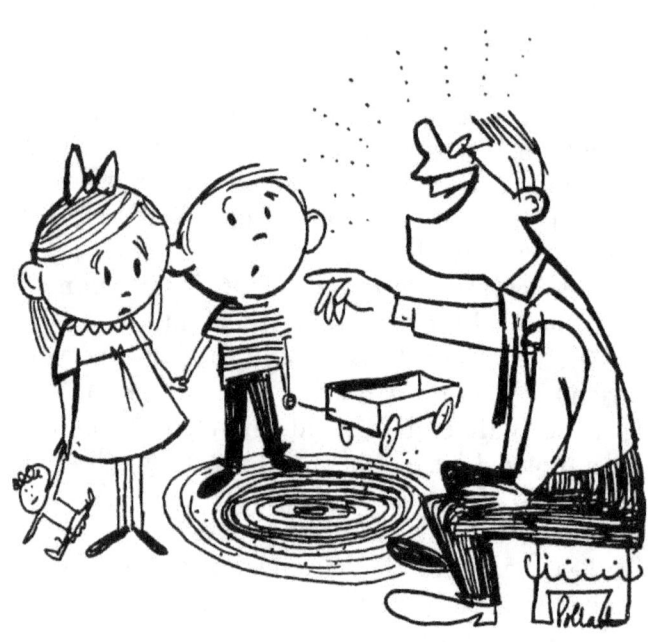

Children who are continually teased about "boy friends' or "girl friends" may come to feel strange about playing and associating with all playmates of the opposite sex.

of course, hinders comfortable, wholesome feelings toward others. It makes children self-conscious and ill poised. And when such feelings continue, they may seriously color a person's attitude to the extent that as an adult he may have difficulty associating or working with men and women of the opposite sex.

But there is one additional facet to the problem of teasing. It does not build a good relationship between the child and the parent (or other person) who teases him. It throws up a barrier between them. The resentment may be silent, yet strong — and needless.

All in fun? Yes, most teasing is considered a harmless little pastime. But children's feelings are real. And wise parents will consider the consequences. Feeling comfortable and right with children of the opposite sex and maintaining a happy relationship between parents and child, is an integral part of sex education. It should not be ignored.

Facts about Masturbation

For generations the very word "masturbation" brought fear and shame. Parents were filled with anxiety when they found their children were involved in what they thought was a shocking and disastrous habit. Children were often frightened and some were even emotionally harmed by the threats of the dreadful results of masturbation. Many of today's parents want the facts. Here are the questions they ask:

Do Many Children Masturbate? Almost all children masturbate to some extent. It is common and natural for children to discover the pleasant sensations which come from pressing against, rubbing or handling the genital organs. In its milder forms, masturbation is not serious and is to be accepted for what it is, a normal part of the growing up experience. Masturbation is most common between the ages of two and six years, and again between the ages of twelve and twenty. However, it may occur at any age.

Why Do Children Masturbate? Many times masturbation is no more than a part of a child's inquisitiveness about his own body. And it usually passes over without any ill effects or difficulties when other interests present themselves to his inquiring mind. On the other hand, some children resort to masturbation in an effort to compensate for a lack of love and affection — something so necessary for the development of healthy minds and bodies. Some children masturbate because they are stimulated by tight clothing. Still others develop the habit during and following chaffing and itching of the skin.

What Damage Is Caused by Masturbation? There is *no* evidence that masturbation causes any physical damage other than an occasional local irritation of the genital area. It does not bring on mental illness, weak eyes, insanity or any other frightening result. Mild masturbation in children is not at all abnormal; it does not cause sexual maladjustment, impotence or sterility. It is not homosexuality. The real injury comes from the anxiety and worry it causes the parents — and then, the child.

What Should Parents Do When a Child Masturbates? In order to help children, parents must first recognize masturbation for what it is — a normal part of "growing up." Infrequent acts of masturbation should be ignored. This is not easy to do when one has been taught that masturbation causes all sorts of dreadful things. But try your best to accept the fact that there is no physical basis for being afraid or worried. Your *attitude* will more than likely determine the end results.

DO NOT threaten your child with punishment. Do not embarrass him or condemn him by saying:

"People won't like you" . . . "such a dirty thing to do!" . . . or "nice children don't do that." Do not frighten him by saying that he will get sick or become infected. Do not offer him rewards in order to make him stop masturbating.

DO look at your child's play life. Does he have plenty of physical activity? Does he have companions his own age? Does he have plenty of play time? Does he have appropriate play things — things he can build, push, pull and handle in his own way? If he is older, does he have a hobby — interests outside of the home? Does he feel accepted, loved and appreciated? If you can answer "yes" to most of these questions there is little likelihood that masturbation will ever become a serious problem with your child.

DO look for other possible causes. Do his clothes fit properly? Is his body clean? Does he have a skin irritation?

Should Parents Talk about Masturbation with Their Children? When a child becomes five or six years old, do not hesitate to talk with him about physically handling himself. It should not turn into a time of embarrassment for him. Simply tell him: "People do not think it looks nice to touch yourself that way. We just don't do it." Let him know that you are not scolding. Be sure that as you discuss it with him, you do it in a calm, relaxed manner. Tell him that all children touch themselves at some time or another; this will help him realize that he is not strange or unusual. Assure him that you know he will not want to do this anymore.

Although "talking it over" may help, it is probably not the best way to control masturbation. If you keep your child occupied and happy, the chances are that the masturbation problem will take care of itself.

What Should Be Done When a Child Masturbates Excessively? Children who masturbate a great deal are usually troubled and unhappy. These are often children who are without friends and who lack a normal amount of childhood fun. In such children masturbation is not the cause of their problem, but the symptom —the warning signal that things are not well in every area of the child's life. So if your child has this problem, cheek to see what is troubling him. Make a definite effort to create good play situations. Does he enjoy active play? Is he provided with worth-while tasks at home? Above all, is he loved and complimented for his accomplishments? He needs to be included in family projects and family fun. But if after you have completed the whole check list he still does not respond, then it is time to seek professional guidance, preferably from a Christian.

"Bad" Language

Stevie ran in the back door with a newly learned word —a really offensive one. Half giggling, he blurted it out and waited for his mother's reaction.

"What do you do at a time like that?" Stevie's mother asks.

To ignore it and behave as though the youngster's word is nothing unusual does not solve the problem. Even a child knows that calm indifference is not a logical reaction. The young offender should know that you realize what he has said. He should know that you understand its meaning. It makes the word less exciting when he discovers you have heard it before!

What should you say? Simply tell him that people consider such language bad manners and unpleasant. Tell him that Jesus does not want him to talk that way. Nothing is ever gained by showing anger or by acting horrified. But youngsters *do* learn from your matter-of-fact disapproval that some expressions are not suitable.

But do not be discouraged if Junior's experimentation with words has reoccurrences — even though you talk with him about it. Trying out bathroom talk, sex words and crude jokes is a stage that many children pass through. However, children who are happy with varied activities usually get bored with such talk before it becomes a problem.

Two-and three-year-olds often repeat toilet words just because they are the ones they know —words they can say with a jingly rhythm. Overlooking them or minimizing them helps these words to disappear. And soon Junior is repeating another "new" word over and over again. And in all probability, this word will be acceptable.

Sometimes a parent may think that a child is being naughty when he says a "bad" word, but actually he may have little or no idea what he has said. Young children learn by mimicking — they add to their vocabulary by repeating new words when they hear them. So if a child picks up an objectionable word from a playmate or a neighbor, it's only natural that he'll try it out for size.

There are several things that can be done to counteract this. Explain to the child in a kind way that some words are not good and we do not say them. Do not make an issue of it because most likely it is not that big an incident to him. Then, as far as possible, check your child's playmates. This is important. Children learn from each other. And it does him no good to be constantly exposed to vulgar language. If he associates with those who talk right, he will talk right, too.

Older children have different reasons for using offensive words and phrases. Sometimes it is a crude attempt at being funny. Occasionally it is a youngster's bid for attention. Boys are especially given to using "bad" language. Often, a boy feels it is necessary to know such words and to use them in order to be accepted as a part of the "gang" or to establish himself as a "big shot." Parents can help a youngster at this stage if they will praise him for the acceptable, "grown-up" things he does. But probably the most effective antidote to combat undesirable language is to pray with him about it. When a child learns that such behavior is displeasing to the Lord, it takes on a different meaning. And as you discuss the problem with him, point out what the Bible has to say about such things: "But shun profane and vain babblings: for they will increase unto more ungodliness" (II Tim. 2:16).

Helping Children Accept Their Roles

Proper sex education helps boys to become manly. And it makes girls feel right and happy about being girls. This is important. People often say, "Boys will be boys; and girls will be girls!" But it really isn't that simple. In a sense some boys don't become men and some girls don't become women. They act and react like the opposite sex. Authorities claim that over two million people in America do *not* accept themselves as they are — their sex role. These unfortunate sex deviates were undoubtedly not born that way. Parents, teachers and other adults caused them to turn to unnatural patterns. So it is not enough to "let nature take its course." Guidance into normal sex roles is important.

Although boys and girls *are* different, it is not a clear-cut difference that allows us to say, "This is just for boys/' and "This is only for girls." Parents who are determined to make their boys out-and-out "he-men" and their girls "real ladies" are on unreasonable territory if they are too rigid in their thinking. Such parents frequently say: "Boys don't play with those things." "That is not a girl's game." "Don't be a sissy; boys don't cry." "That's too hard for a girl to do." Statements like these usually tell

79

us more about the parents than they do about the children.

The truth of the matter is that men do cry sometimes, women do enjoy athletics, and although men usually work away from the home, women frequently

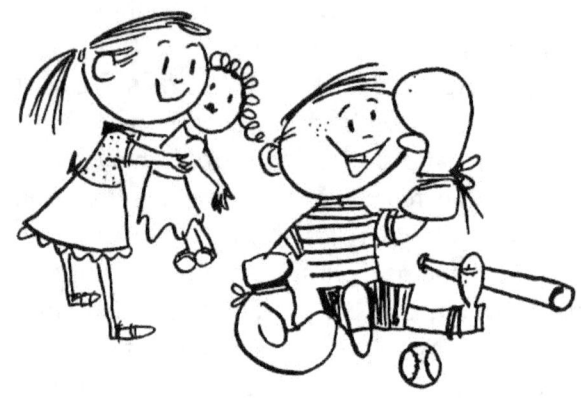

It is hard for a child to accept his own sex if his parents keep wishing he were different.

do, too. Since boys and girls are first of all *people,* they are more alike than they are different. There is much overlapping of masculine and feminine activities. So let your youngster develop his own interests within the wide range of what is acceptable and normal. Your child is a unique person and he needs to grow into the kind of person he really is. Undoubtedly children benefit from associating with both men and women. Youngsters who associate almost exclusively with one sex are at a disadvantage in knowing what the other is like.

It is unwise to force a child toward an unnatural sex pattern. He should be encouraged to develop into his own normal sex role —without the disapproval or regret of his parents. Francis' parents, for example, longed for a girl. There were already four boys at home. And then the doctor announced, "Another bouncing baby boy!" His parents were disappointed. And they showed their disappointment by often casting Francis into a girl's role. In fact, he soon learned that if he were to live up to his mother's expectations, he would have to play the part of a girl. This was the unfortunate beginning of a long history that finally led to sex deviation.

It is hard for a child to accept his own sex if his parents keep wishing he were different. He finds it difficult being himself. All too often such boys are over-protected, over-dressed and frequently handed a girl's part. And girls who live in such an environment are pressured into male interests, masculine dress and boyish hair styles.

If you want your child to adjust happily to his sex, you should lovingly accept him for what he is. As a psychologist I am occasionally called upon to counsel with homosexuals — adults who are inordinately attracted to their own sex. In nearly every case they have had parents who through the years caused them to be dissatisfied with their own sex.

Parents have the important responsibility of helping a boy feel proudly masculine; of encouraging a little girl to be sweetly feminine. This is best accomplished without undue pressure. In a home where the father fills his God-assigned role as the understanding head of the family, young sons naturally sense their part in the scheme of things-to-come. A mother's loving cooperation as the homemaker sets the stage for a small daughter to find her place. Such God-planned living lays solid foundations for future happiness in human relationships, including marriage.

Should a Child Be Given Books about Sex?

There is an old saying, "Books are our best teachers." And of course books are good teachers, but they cannot take the place of a *person*.

A friendly, comfortable conversation that discusses *your youngsters* questions is better than any book. Printed materials give facts, and many of them do it in a natural, positive manner. But it is the author's way, not timed to your child's thinking. A youngster asks his questions when he becomes curious about some particular thing, and it is not easy to use a book to answer what is on a child's mind without getting into other information. And this additional information is often beyond his present curiosity or understanding.

Books are limited in other ways, too. They are impersonal. They cannot create the warm, friendly, wholesome attitude that loving parents can. And this "just right" attitude is one of the most important parts of sex education. In a quiet, subtle way it tells your child that sex is a part of living. He learns to accept it as something that is wholesome and God-given.

However, there are some parents who find it difficult to talk with their children about matters

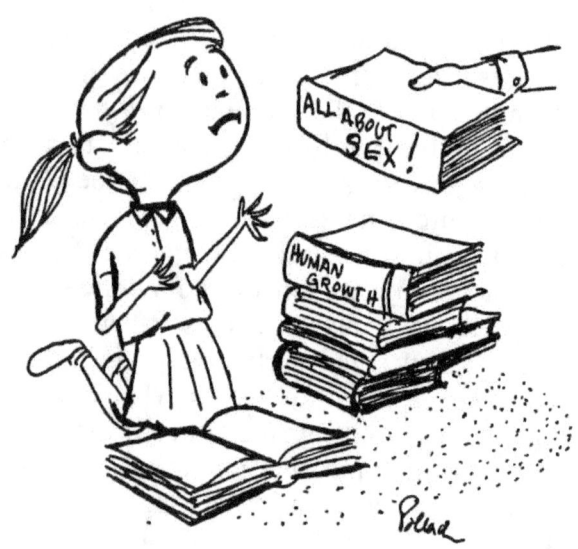

Books are important. But they cannot create the friendly, wholesome attitude that loving parents can.

of sex. When this is true a good book is useful, especially if the parent and the child read the book together. If you are using a book with your youngster, remember to give him plenty of time to say what he thinks and feels. Give him ample opportunity to ask the questions that come to his mind.

Parents can often clarify their own thinking through the aid of a book. It can also be a source where parents can find appropriate answers to the questions their children ask. Your pastor, doctor or librarian can suggest books available in this field. In addition, your Christian bookseller can show you the finest books available.

There are also some excellent books that you can share with your children when a new baby is coming into the family. Written in easy story form, these books help youngsters understand many of the things they need to know about the new baby and the "hows and whys" of his arrival.

As you read books for your own information, as you share books with your child, don't forget: You are the important influence. In years to come it will be *your* actions, *your* feelings and *your* spiritual insights which will take the central position in the attitudes your sons and daughters hold toward sex.

Explaining the Father's Role in Reproduction

"How do you explain the father's role in reproduction?" This is a question nearly all parents ask.

One of the privileges of parenthood is explaining human reproduction to one's children. But the way in which it is presented will affect the children's attitudes for years to come, not only during childhood but also as they enter adolescence, then adulthood. So when parents interpret mating as a wonderful, wholesome process ordained in marriage by God, their children will think of it in the same way.

It is impossible to predict just when a child will ask questions about mating. Each child has his own rate of development. But sometime after five or six, a youngster starts reaching out for greater understandings. He wants to know the reasons why: "What makes my kite fly?" "Why does the cat have whiskers?" "Can fish hear?" There are questions, questions and more questions as he tries to get to the fundamentals, the beginnings. It is only natural for him to ask, "Just how does a baby get started?"

To tell a child about the father's role in reproduction may seem difficult, especially for parents whose childhood training did not include discussion of sex matters. But actually it is easy. And children accept it readily.

Children need to know from the very beginning that every baby has *two* parents. The concept of each baby child and each baby animal having both a mother and a father is important because it paves the way later on for a child to understand the father's part in reproduction. Parents should point out to small children the fact that animals like baby kittens and puppies have both a mother and a father.

When little Judy asks if she can have a baby when she grows up, parents should say, "Yes? when you grow up and get *married* you can have a baby. Each baby needs both a mother and a father."

"It takes a mother and a father to start a baby." This explanation may be enough for awhile, but not for long. In time — possibly between six and nine years of age, the child will want to know just how this comes about. Simply tell him that a cell (or seed, or sperm) from the father must join with a cell (or seed, or egg) in the mother's body. These father and mother cells are so small that you cannot even see them. But after they are joined together, a wonderful thing happens —God causes a baby to start growing. And when the baby has grown big enough, it is born.

Perhaps immediately, perhaps later, your child

will ask, "But how does the father's seed get into the mother?"

Then you can say, "You know how a boy is made — he has a penis. You know that a girl is made differently. She has an opening called a vagina. God planned this difference. He made a man different from a woman so it would be possible for a baby to be started. God planned it in such a way that the father's penis can fit into the mother's vagina. The tiny little seed (called semen) flows from the father's penis into the mother. This is the way all babies are started. And it is God's way for a little new life to begin."

It is important that your child know the difference between semen and urine. Explain to him that semen is not urine; it is quite different, and is especially made to carry the sperm from the father's body.

Parents realize that any answer they give their children concerning sexual intercourse leaves much unexplained because a child cannot understand the deep feelings involved. These understandings will come to him as he grows older.

The answers he needs at this time must be ones that make sense when they are added to the facts he has been given before. He needs truthful answers, ones which give the father's role its rightful importance in the family picture.

But be sure that *love* is a vital part of the story. Tell of the love a mother and father have for each other. Speak of the fact that they *want* a baby to love. And of course, actions speak louder than words. Youngsters become capable of receiving and expressing love when they are loved themselves — when their parents create a family life of warmth and affection. And when a child has been reared in an atmosphere of love, he senses the fact that love is an integral part of sex.

It is easy for a child to accept the father's part in the wonderful story of fertilization when his daddy has been a comforter, a story reader and an excursion engineer as well as a disciplinarian. In homes where both parents lovingly work out family problems and plan the family fun, children are quick to say, "Of course we need *two* parents. Daddies are important, and fun, too!"

These, then, are the natural steps in explaining the father's part in reproduction: (1) Every baby has a mother and a father, (2) God has wonderfully planned it this way, (3) sexual relations are the result of the mother and father loving each other so much, and (4) give a simple explanation of mating.

When Children Ask
about Menstruation

Children may ask about menstruation at any age. Just leafing through a magazine, or helping with the grocery shopping may make a child wonder about such things. "What is this?" he asks, pointing to a well-advertised box.

Here again your answers must be truthful and also geared to the child's level of understanding. The complex chemistry of menstruation is beyond young children. But they are satisfied with a simple explanation.

Here is an explanation of menstruation that is helpful to boys and girls who are approximately nine years of age. Tell the child that while a baby is growing inside of the mother it cannot get its food by eating as we do —so God made it possible for the baby to be fed from the mother's blood. Even when there is no baby growing, a supply of blood collects each month in a special place inside of the mother just to be ready if a baby does start. If no baby begins to grow, then this blood is not needed and it is discharged through the mother's vagina. This happens each month to all grown women. It is called menstruation. It is like bleeding — but not due to a cut or hurt. God made ladies like that; and that's the way they are *supposed* to

90

be. It is part of God's plan to always have fresh blood and proper food ready for a new baby whenever it begins to grow.

"Does it hurt to menstruate?" children want to know. You can point out that many women do not feel any pain or discomfort at all, while others may feel a little tired and they may not have their usual pep. But almost all women are perfectly able to go right ahead with their everyday activities. As you speak about menstruation be careful to avoid words which suggest pain —like "cramps," "being sick" and "the curse." Such words are unwisely used. When you call menstruation by its right name, you will help your child to know that it is normal and not to be feared.

Sometimes children ask, "Do men menstruate?" Remind your child that menstruation is just the body's way of throwing away blood that is not needed because there is no baby growing inside the mother. Since men never have babies, of course they do not menstruate.

Make certain your girls have a thorough knowledge of the whys and hows of menstruation before they enter their teens. To menstruate without understanding what is taking place can be a frightening experience.

And remember, the process of menstruation is just as important to boys as it is to girls. It gives boys a greater respect for womanhood and it helps them to understand their sisters and mother —as well as girl friends.

91

The Preadolescent and His Questions

"What's happened to Johnny?" ask many parents of a ten- or eleven-year-old. They remember the happy, busy Johnny of a year ago, and look with misgivings at the new Johnny. He is often rude, loud and rebellious. He teases and disagrees with almost every adult idea. He doesn't pay attention.

What has happened to Johnny? Nothing too alarming — he's just growing up. And although he isn't exactly enjoyable or lovable during these pre-adolescent years, he is normal. Most youngsters between nine and thirteen have times of restless, unpredictable behavior as they experiment this way and that way with their many new ideas.

Although the new Johnny is hard to live with at times, he is basically the same nice child he was a year or so ago, and he needs understanding and wise guidance in spite of his know-it-all attitude. Fortunately, the preadolescent is a realistic individual, and he is interested in the facts — facts with a touch of the scientific, facts he can check in books. This interest in facts makes him a good subject for sex education — education based on what he wants to know.

Is the preadolescent child interested in sex matters? Sometimes yes, sometimes no. Occasionally it seems that the preadolescent develops a strong and sudden interest in sex. He may try to read everything with a sex flavor that he can find — books, magazine articles and newspaper accounts of criminal sex behavior.

If you have had an easy, friendly relationship with your child during his early years of questionings and all through his year by year development of sex understanding, he will probably come to you with many questions. Some of the questions will seem almost like the questions he asked years ago. Don't make the preadolescent feel self-conscious by saying, "Goodness, I told you that ages ago!" Instead, take the opportunity to give clear, definite explanations. His quick, well-developed mind will have no trouble remembering the terms now. And he will soon fit them into his old understandings of sex matters.

The preadolescent girl wonders — and needs to know:

"When will I menstruate?"

"Why do I have to menstruate anyway?"

"Will I menstruate all my life?"

"What should I do when I begin to menstruate?"

These questions need friendly, correct answers. Menstruation isn't frightening to the girl who understands what it is all about.

A boy has questions, too! He wonders how long it is going to be until he will have to start shaving. He wonders about some of the conversation he hears from certain boys at school. What about girls and menstruation, anyway? If a father and son have had good times and good talks through the growing up years, the boy often feels easier if he can talk these things over with his dad. However, if the mother is handy she may find she is asked questions

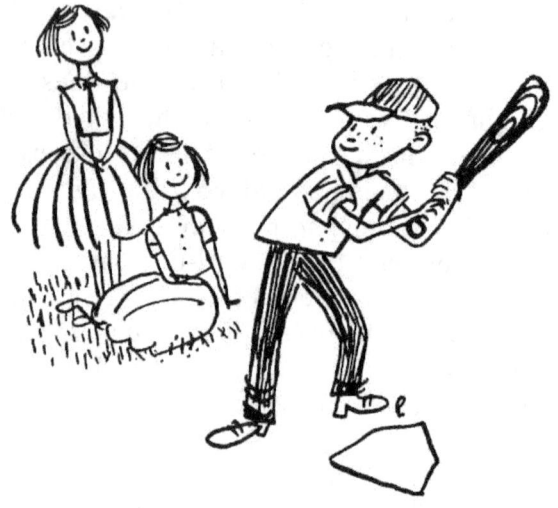

The preadolescent asks many questions similar to those he raised a few years earlier. The clear definite explanations you give him now will help him to become a happy, well poised adult.

by either her son or her daughter. Preadolescents may want to know:

"When do mothers and fathers mate?"

"Does a baby start every time parents mate?" "How do you know when you are going to have a baby?"

"What does the male sperm look like?"

"Is the female egg like a hen's egg?"

"What makes a baby look like its parents?" "What makes a baby a boy or a girl?"

"Boys don't menstruate, do they?"

"What is a wet dream?"

"Do people who aren't married have babies?" Some children have questions but for one reason or another find it difficult to speak about sex matters. If your child is silent don't take for granted that he doesn't wonder. Everyday happenings are good starting places for matter-of-fact information. A family situation, a wedding, a birth or a pregnancy may be a natural opportunity to casually talk things over.

Above all, let your preadolescent child know you love him. Outbursts of temper, arguing and defiance are not unusual with the "almost" grown-up child. Remember that he is full of uncertainties and much wondering. Give him quiet, firm correction when he warrants it, but also flood him with understanding and love. His confidence in your affection is as important as the information you give him. And it will help him gain wholesome, healthy sex attitudes that will help him become a happy, well poised adult.

Safeguarding Your Child

Mary and her mother were hurrying home from the market. But they had only reached the corner when it started to rain. Just then an automobile pulled alongside the curb, and a friendly sounding man called out, "Want a ride?"

"Oh, uh, well, no thank you," replied Mother. "We'll soon be home. Thank you just the same."

As the car drove down the street, Mary looked up at Mother and said, "Mommie, why didn't you let the man take us home?"

"Come, honey," Mother urged. "Let's walk as fast as we can. It *is* raining hard. And as soon as we get home I'll explain about getting into cars with strangers."

Mary's mother handled the situation wisely. We all know that there is a significant number of criminals, sex fiends and other abnormal people who would take advantage of young children and harm them if they had the opportunity.

From the time boys and girls are quite young, they need to know how to protect themselves from individuals who are potentially dangerous. When you warn children about strangers, you should keep three factors in mind: (1) Do not frighten them, but (2) do teach them a healthy respect for strangers and (3) help your children set up some definite safeguards.

You can avoid frightening your child by quietly explaining that most people are good and kind, but some are *not;* and when a person is a stranger you can not always be certain whether he is nice or not.

Here are some rules that you can teach children:

1. Do not go into lonely places by yourself.

2. Do not talk or walk or ride with strangers.

3. Do not stay away from the house after dark.

4. Do not open the door to strangers if you are in the house alone.

5. Do not accept candy or food from strangers.

6. Do tell your mother and father if someone tries to get you to go someplace with him alone.

Try to give these instructions without causing undue fear. However, this is not always easy. Newspapers, magazines, radio and television make sex crimes vivid and frightening to young children. This means that you have the delicate task of reassuring your child that he need not live in fear. "Such cases are unusual/" you should tell him. But at the same time it is necessary to make and enforce rules that will protect your child from the "unusual."

One of the most important guides for your child is your own friendly reserve with strangers. Since ideas are "caught" as well as "taught," he will soon develop a natural reserve around strangers — a bearing that will be one of his *best safeguards.*

Also available from www.sunvillagepublications.com

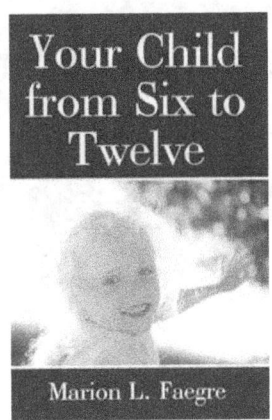

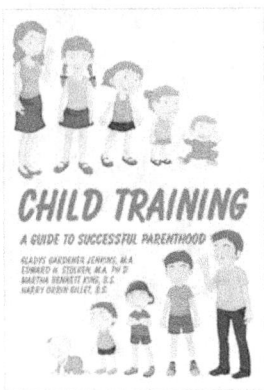

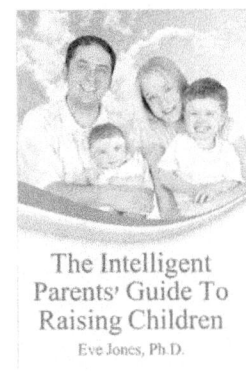

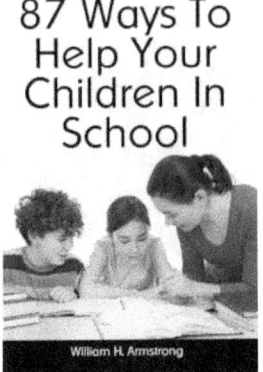

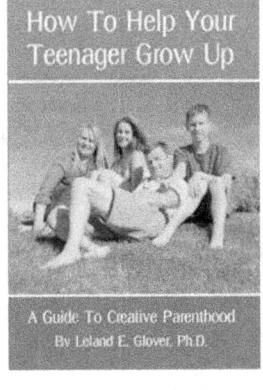

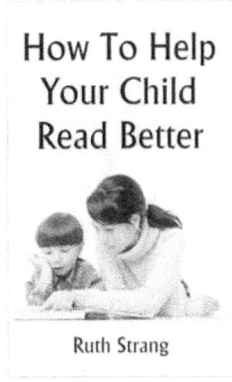

How To Teach Children
The Joy of Reading

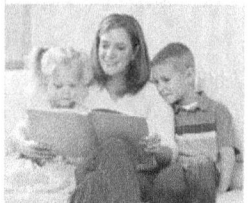

A Guide for Parents and Teachers

Ellen C. Henderson

**Launching
Your
Preschooler**

How To Help Make Your Child's
First Experiences A Breeze!

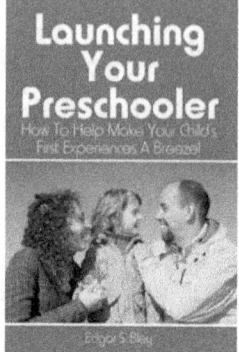

Edgar S. Bley

HOW TO PREVENT
STUTTERING IN
CHILDREN

A Guide for Parents and Teachers

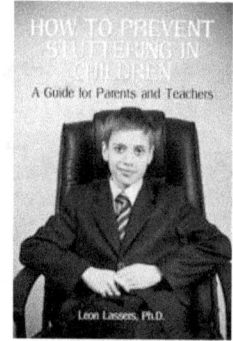

Leon Lassers, Ph.D.

Teach Your
Child To Talk

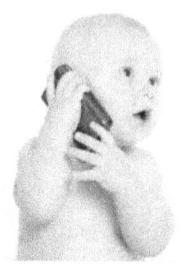

How To Tell
Children
About Sex

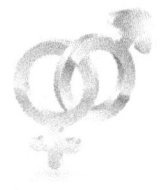

Clyde M. Narramore, Ed.D.